I NEVER DREAMED I WOULD BE A SUPER COOL BARBER BUT HERE I AM

My Coloring Lab

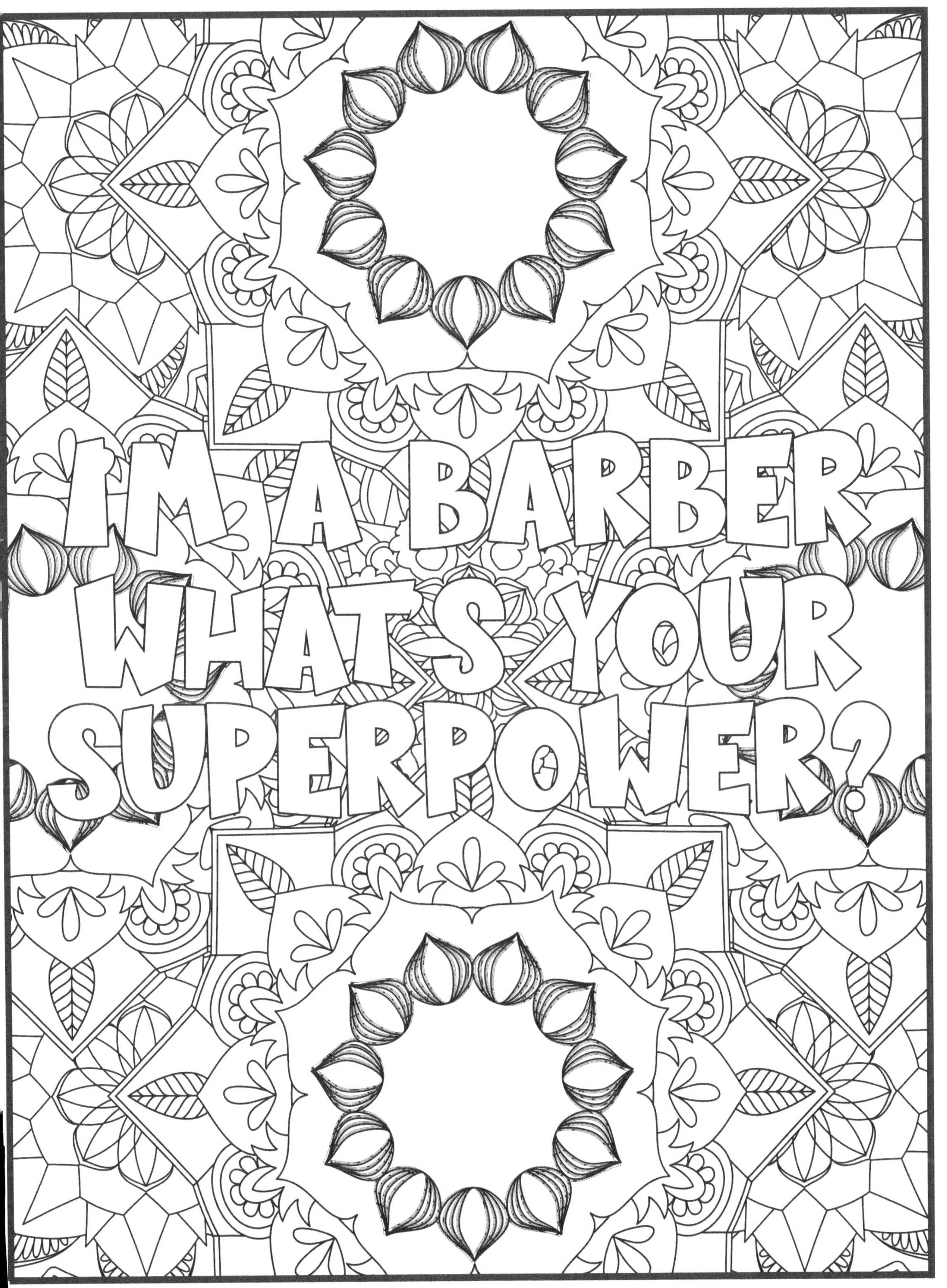

I'M A BARBER WHAT'S YOUR SUPERPOWER?

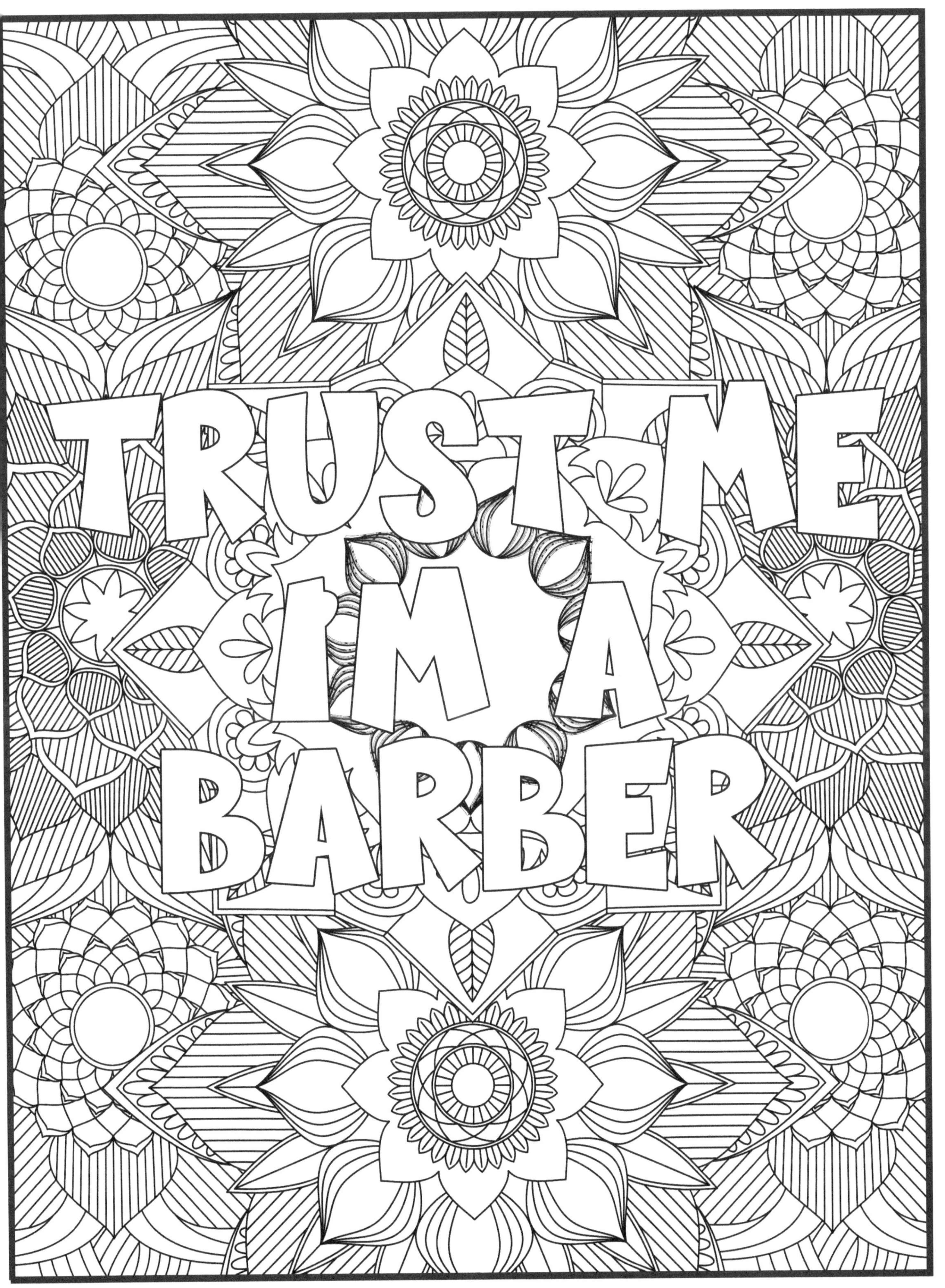
TRUST ME
I'M A
BARBER

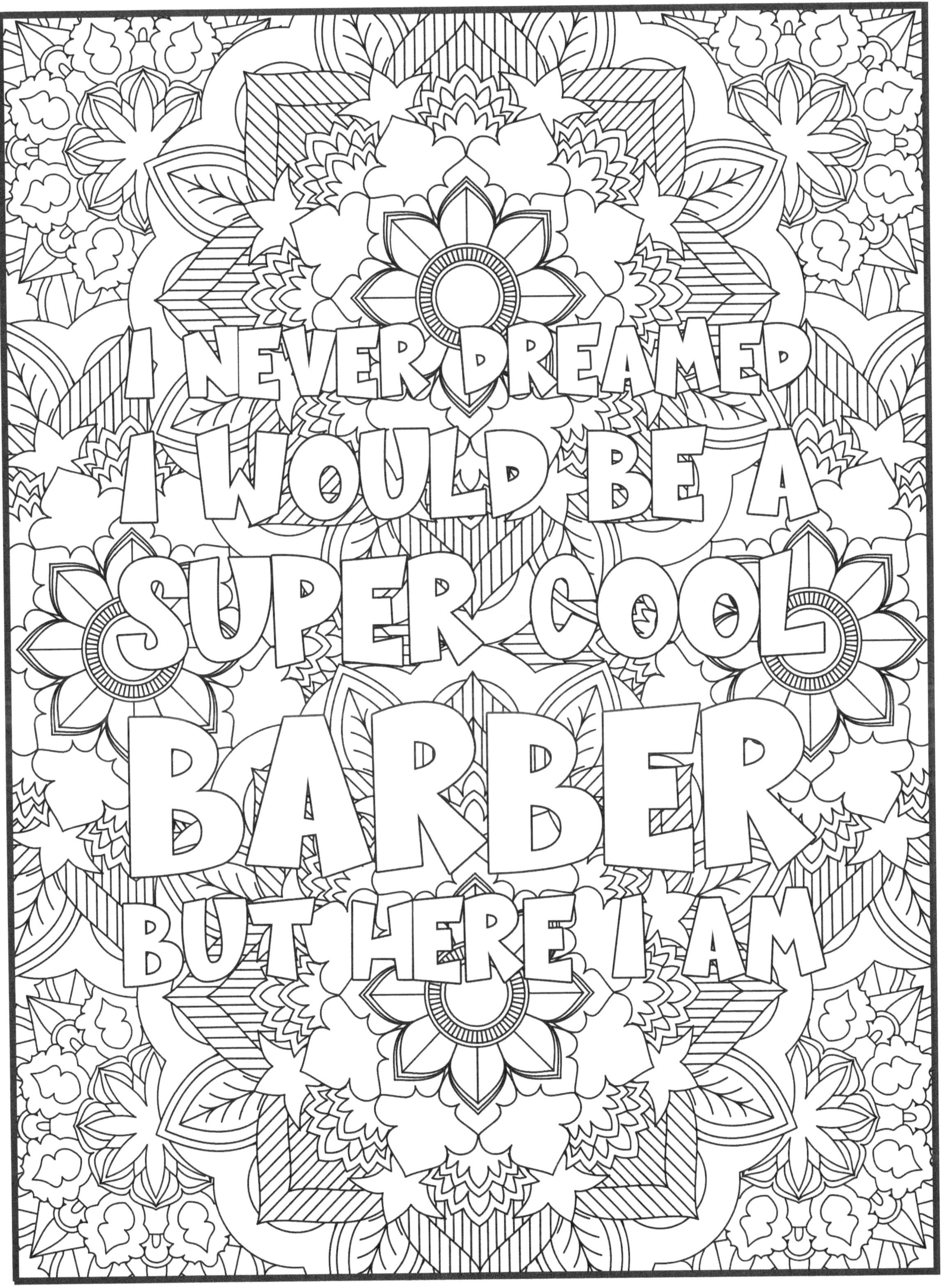

I NEVER DREAMED
I WOULD BE A
SUPER COOL
BARBER
BUT HERE I AM

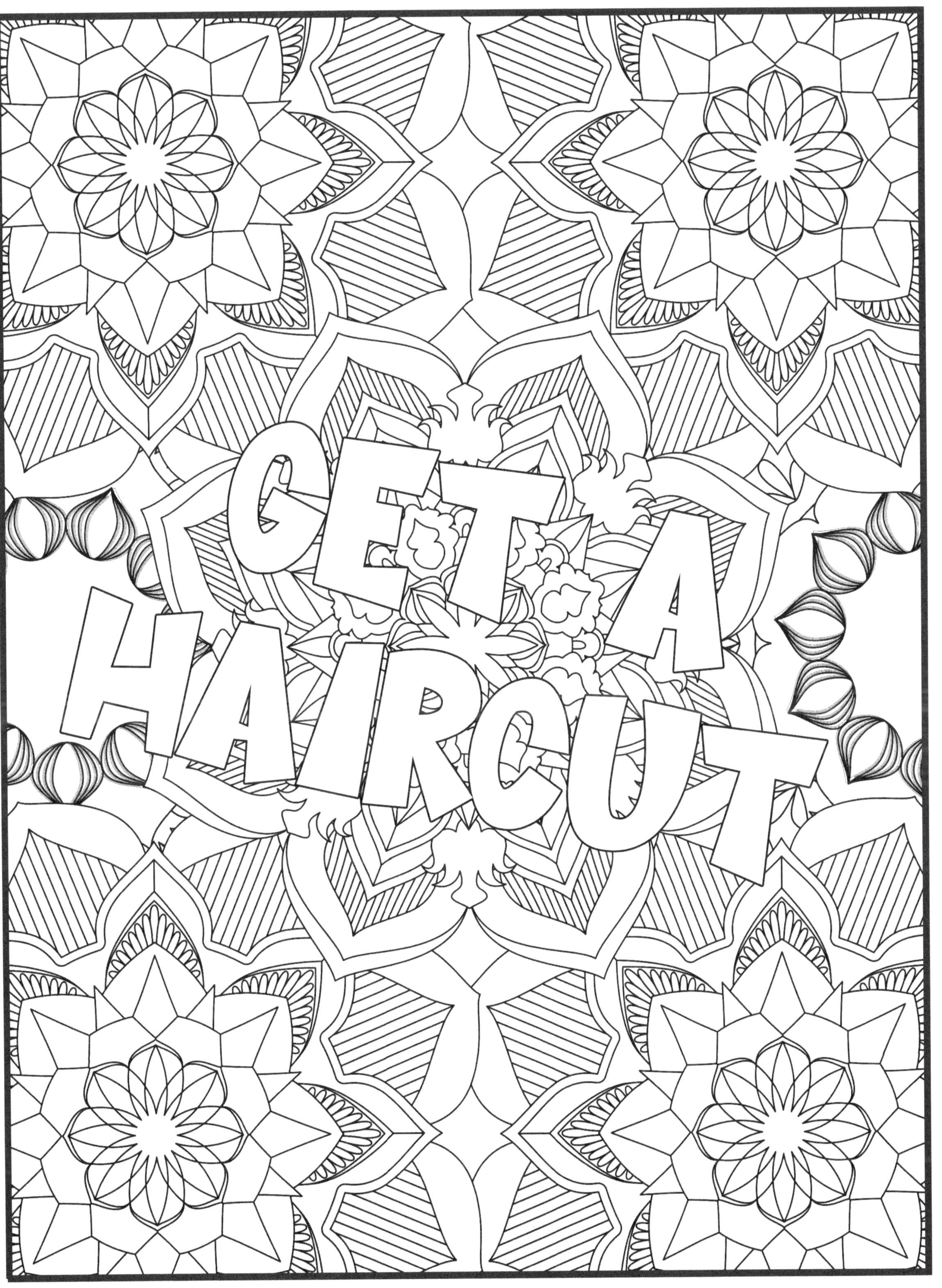

GET A HAIRCUT

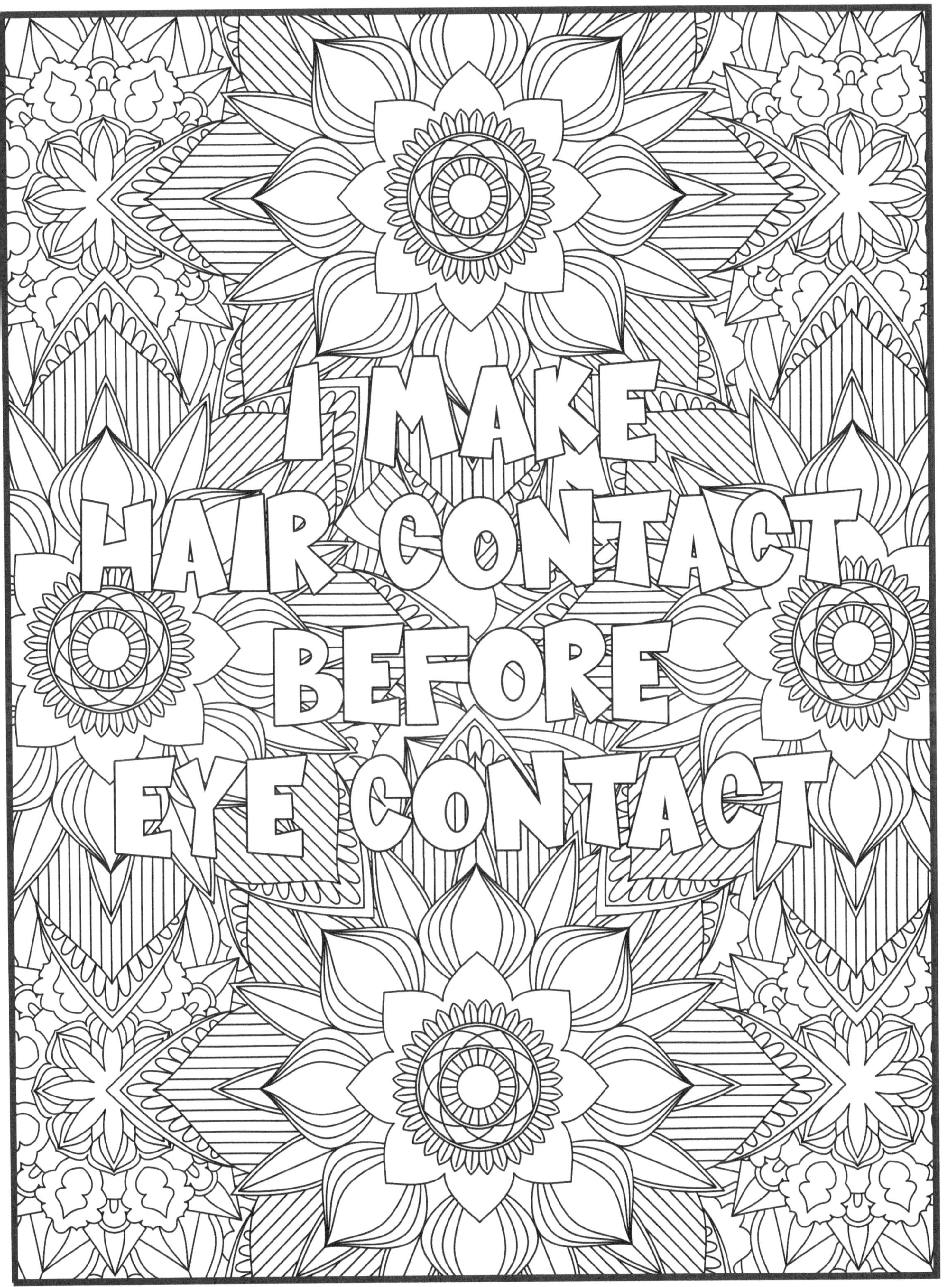

I MAKE
HAIR CONTACT
BEFORE
EYE CONTACT

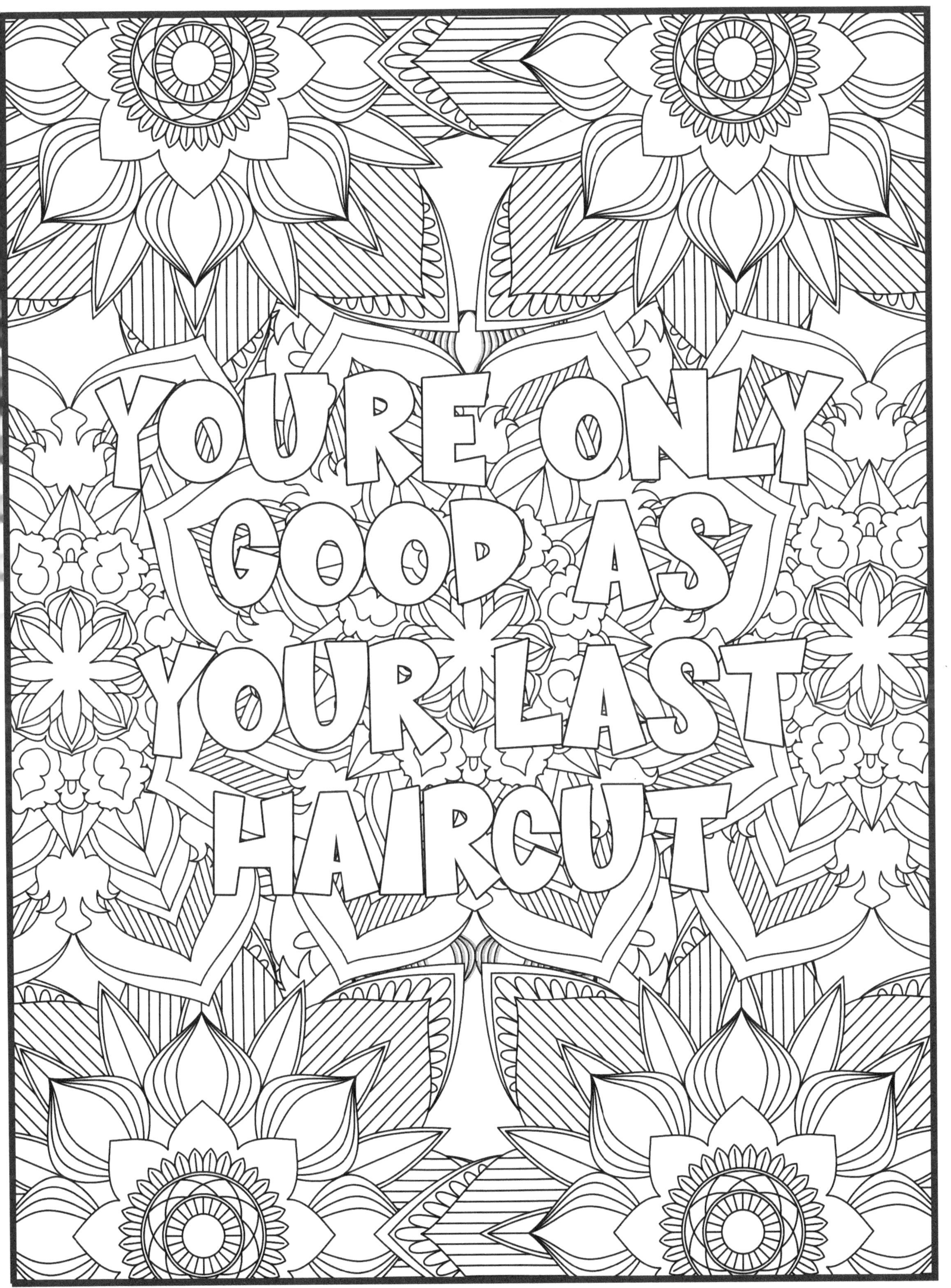

YOU'RE ONLY
GOOD AS
YOUR LAST
HAIRCUT

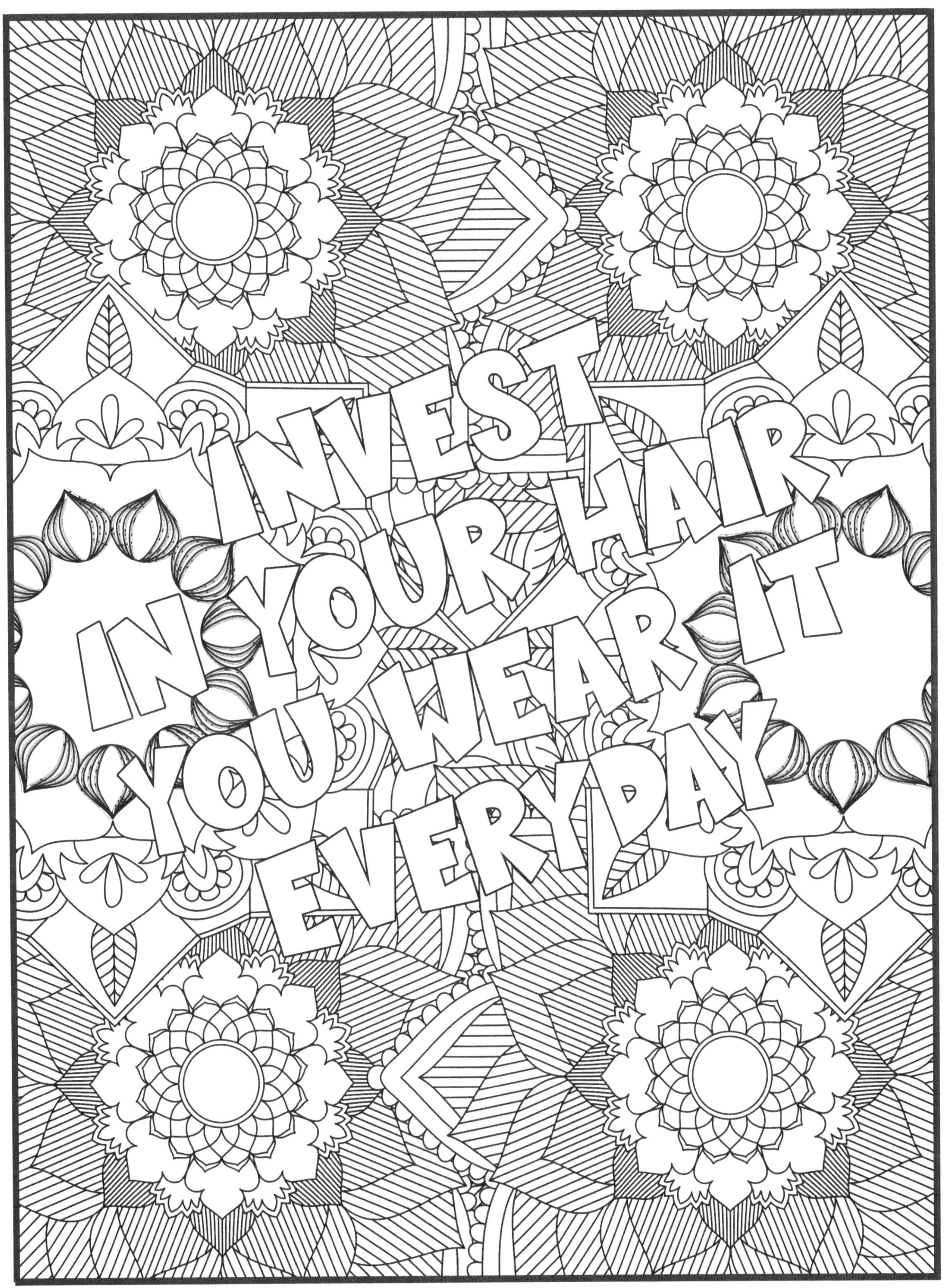

INVEST
IN YOUR HAIR
YOU WEAR IT
EVERYDAY

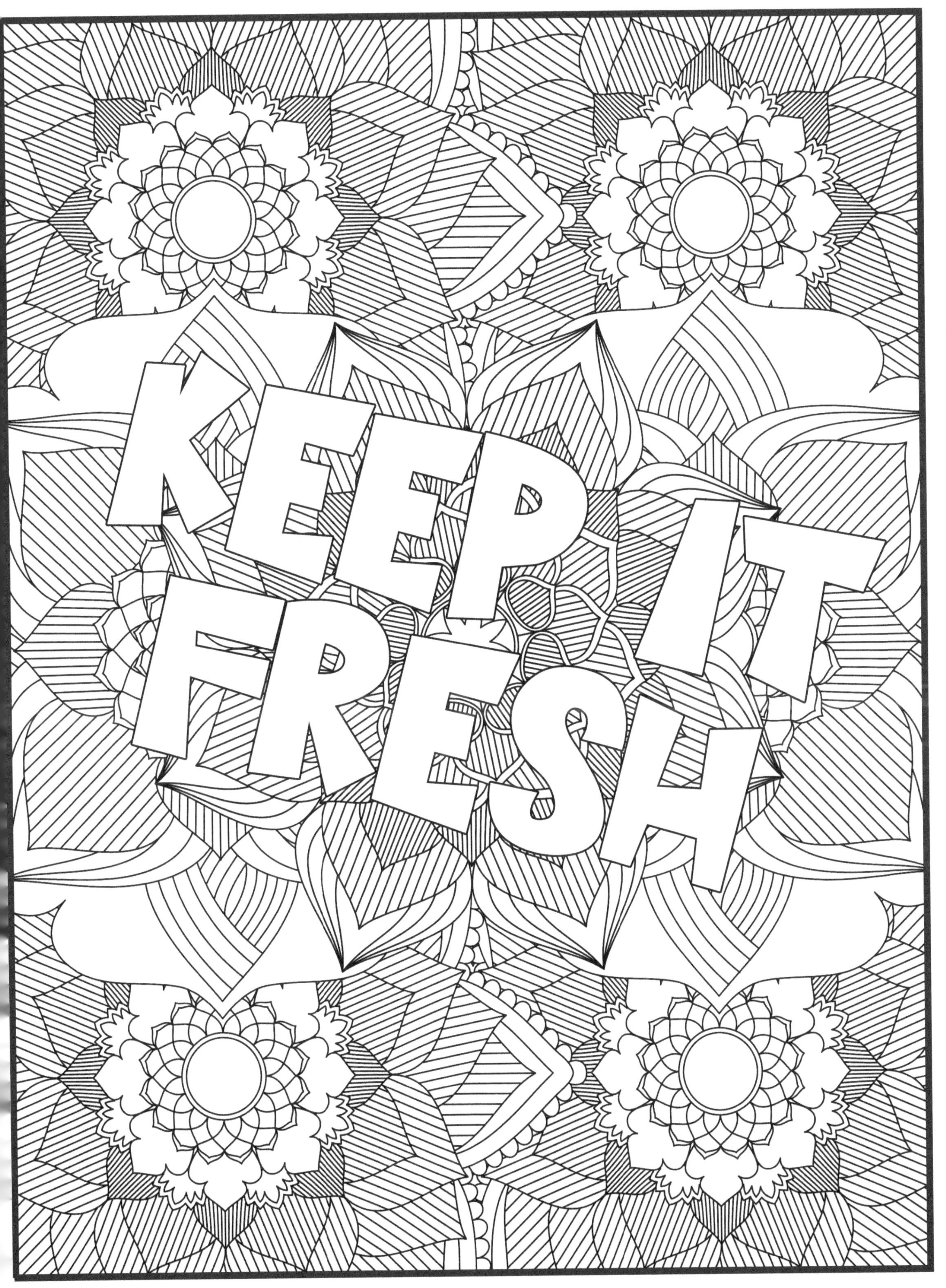

KEEP IT FRESH

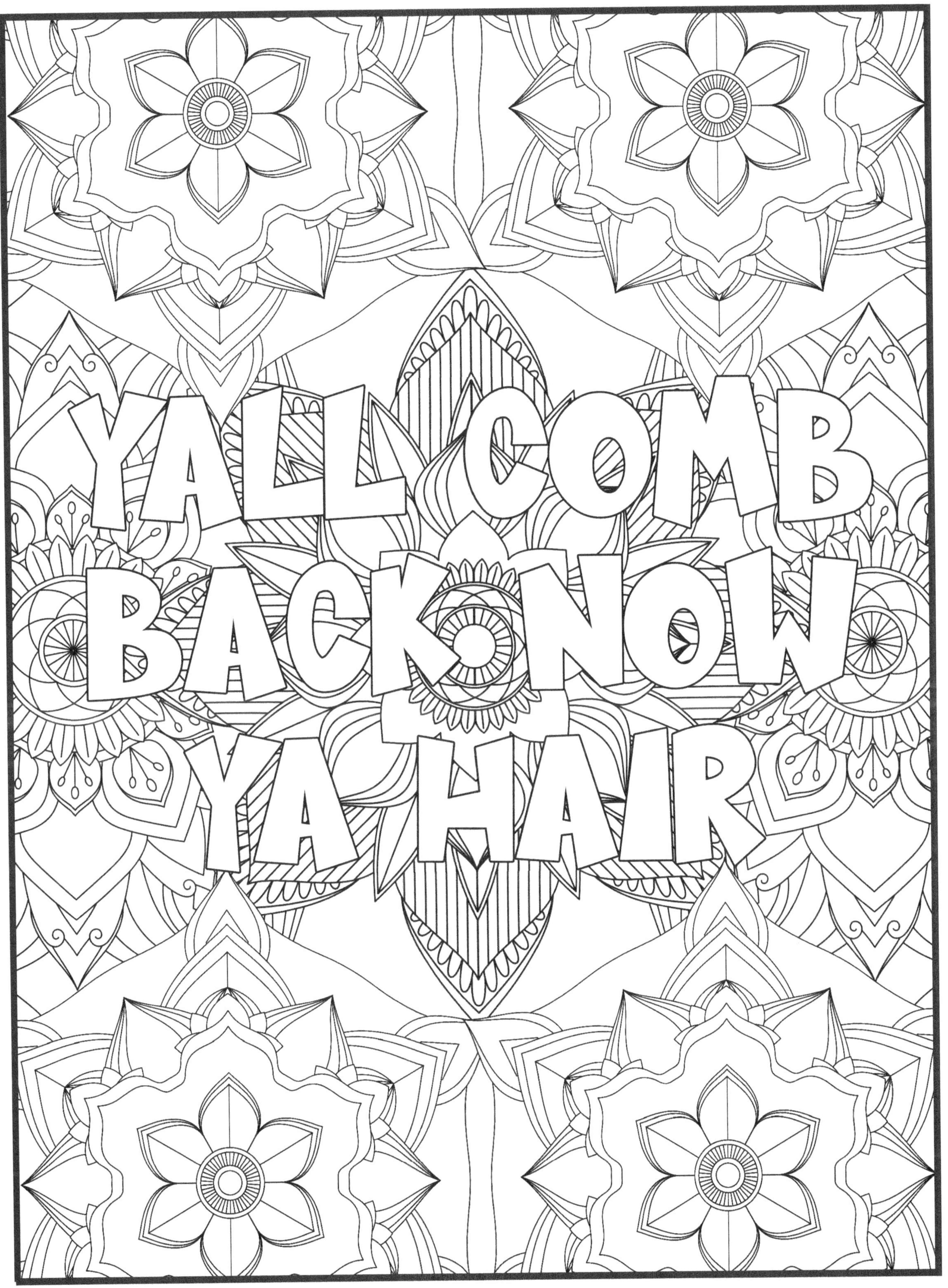

YALL COMB
BACK NOW
YA HAIR

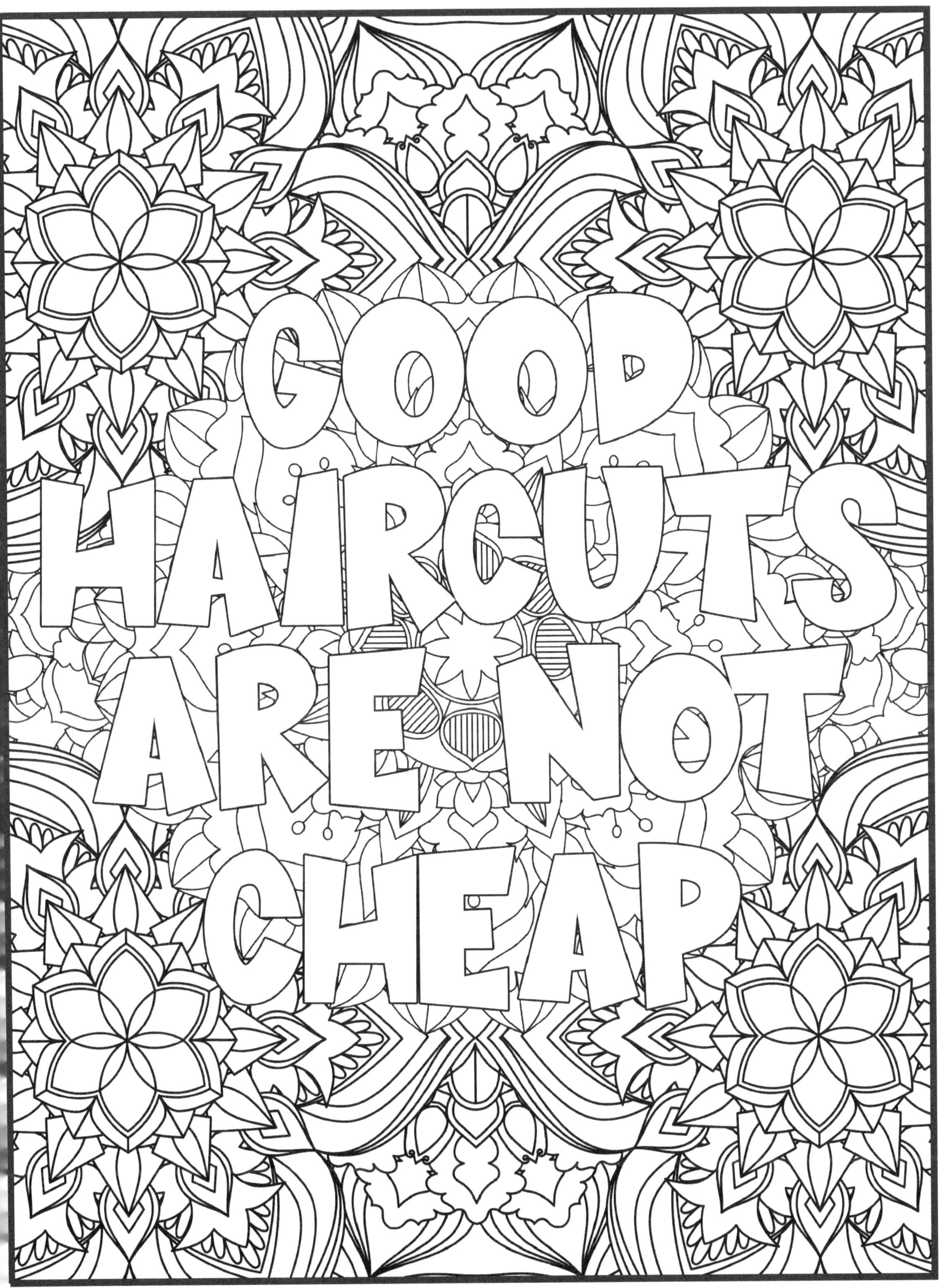

GOOD
HAIRCUTS
ARE NOT
CHEAP

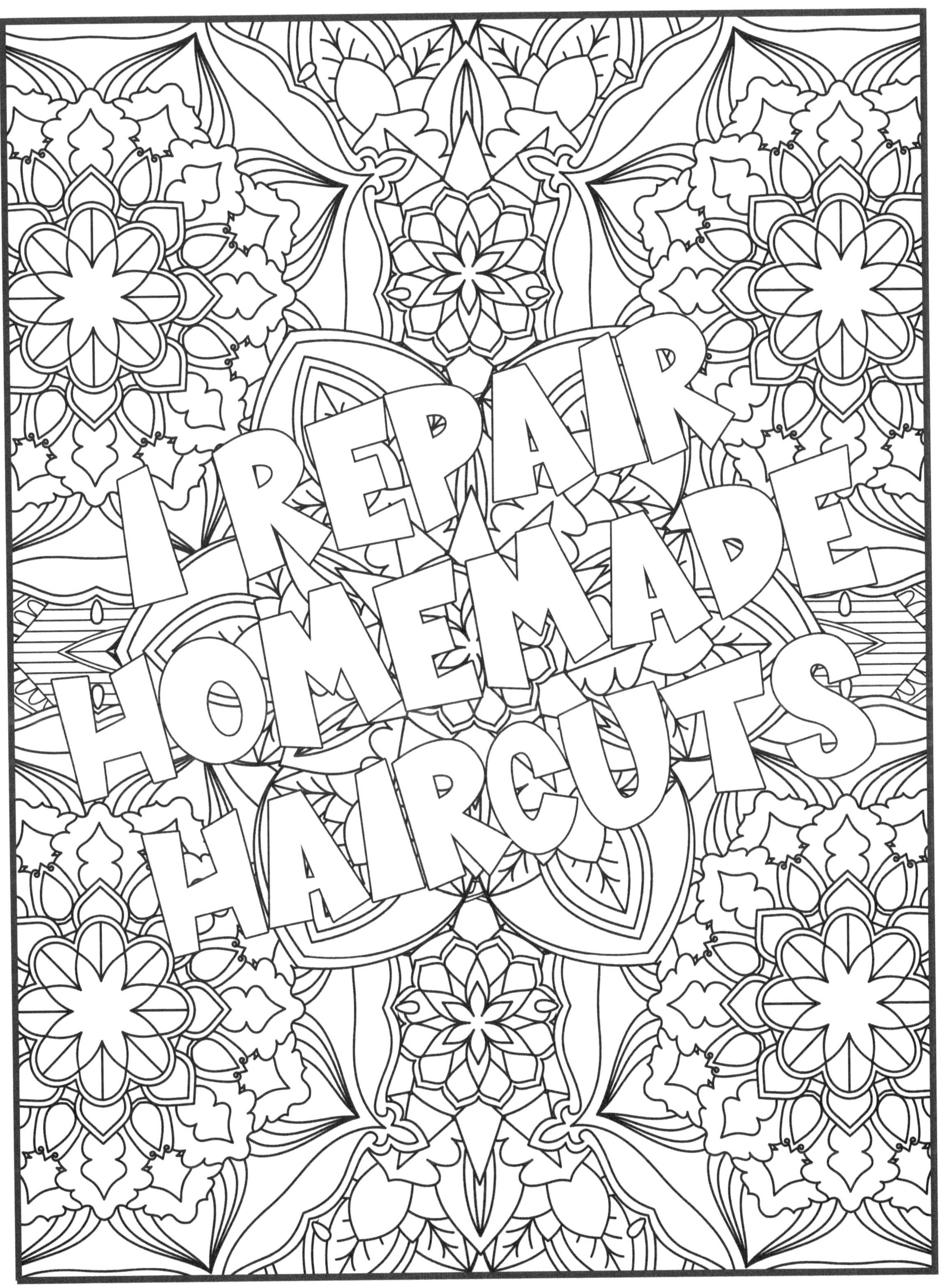
I REPAIR
HOMEMADE
HAIRCUTS

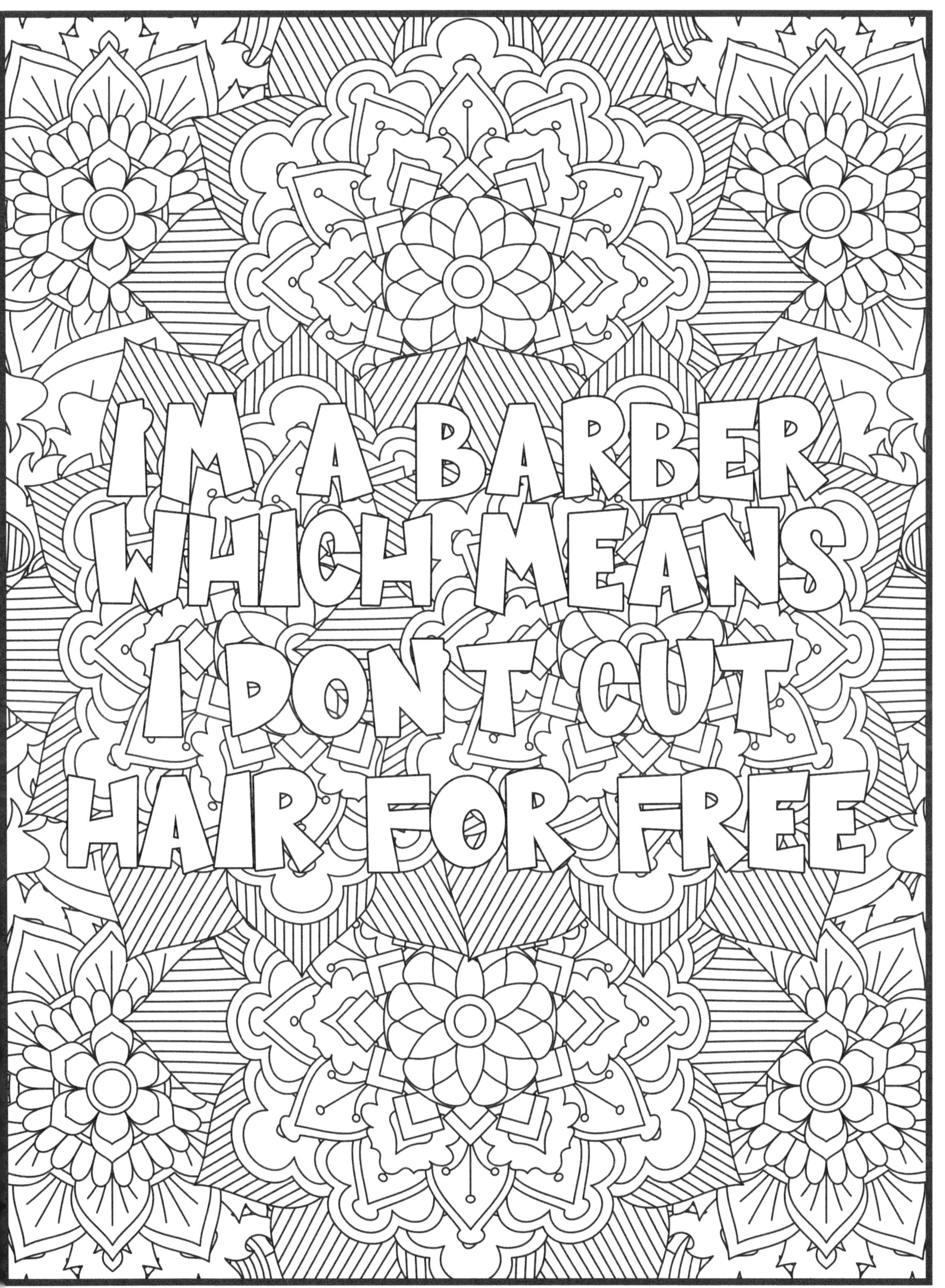

IM A BARBER WHICH MEANS I DON'T CUT HAIR FOR FREE

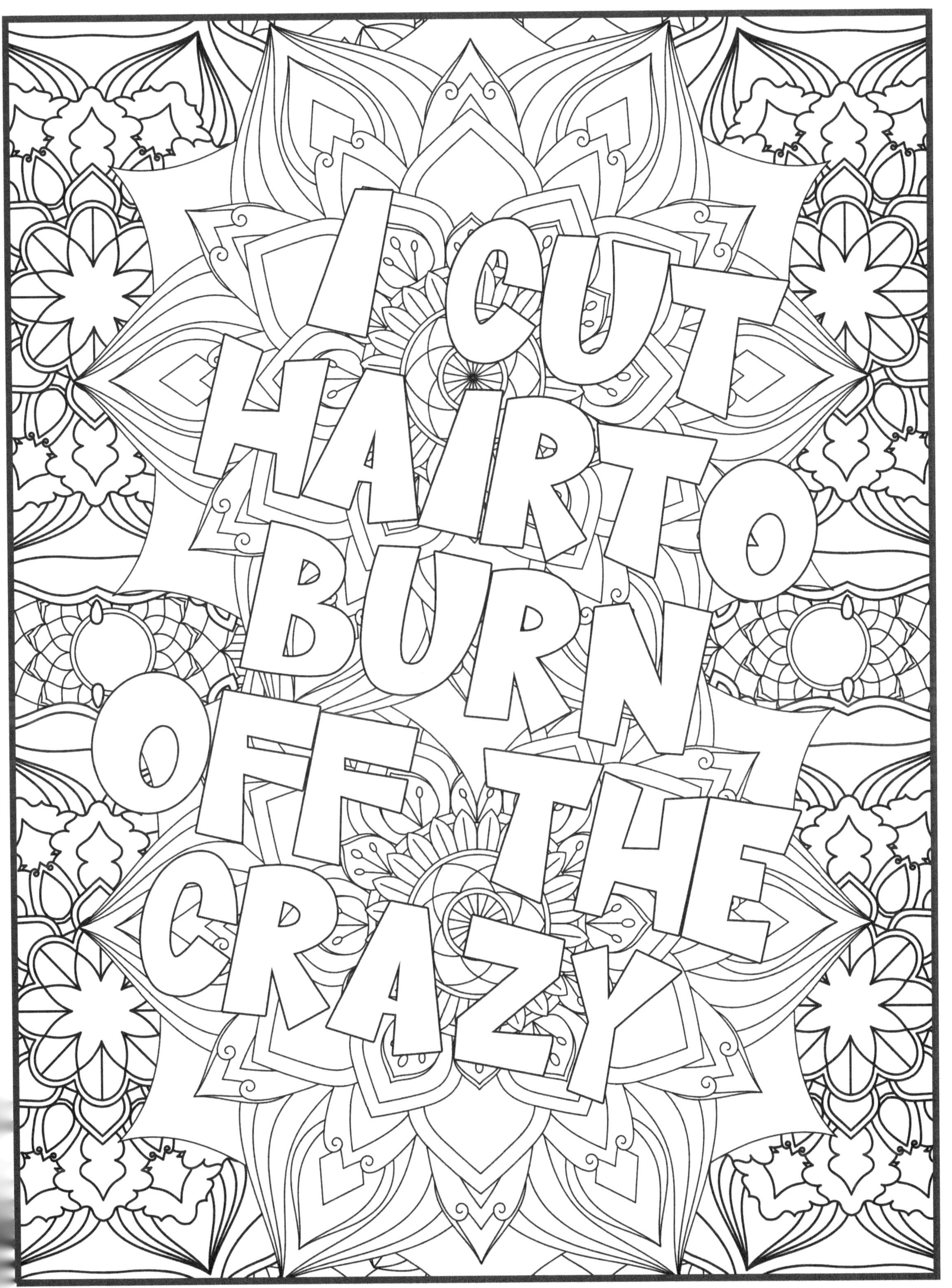

I CUT
HAIR TO
BURN
OFF THE
CRAZY

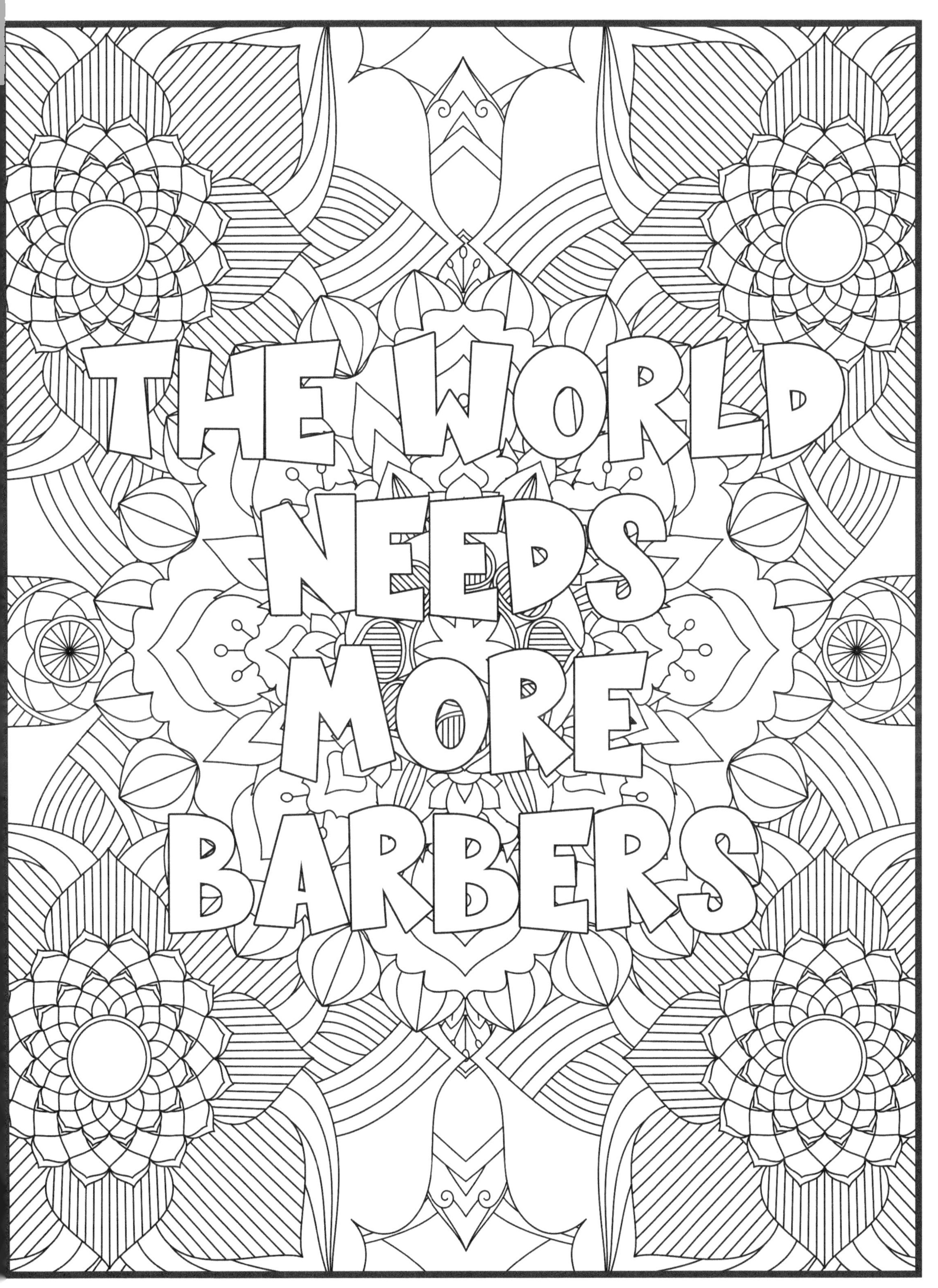

THE WORLD
NEEDS
MORE
BARBERS

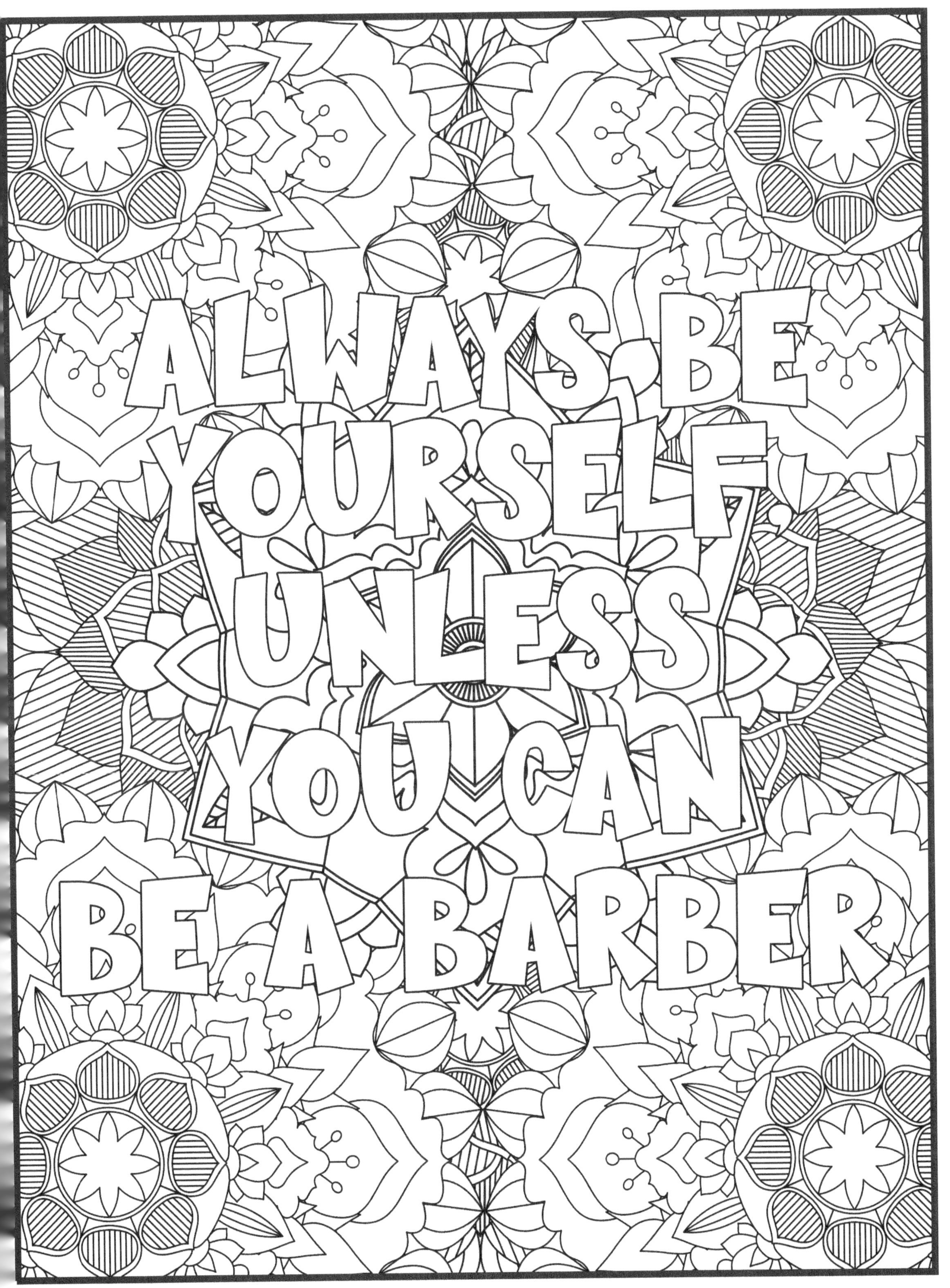

ALWAYS BE
YOURSELF
UNLESS
YOU CAN
BE A BARBER

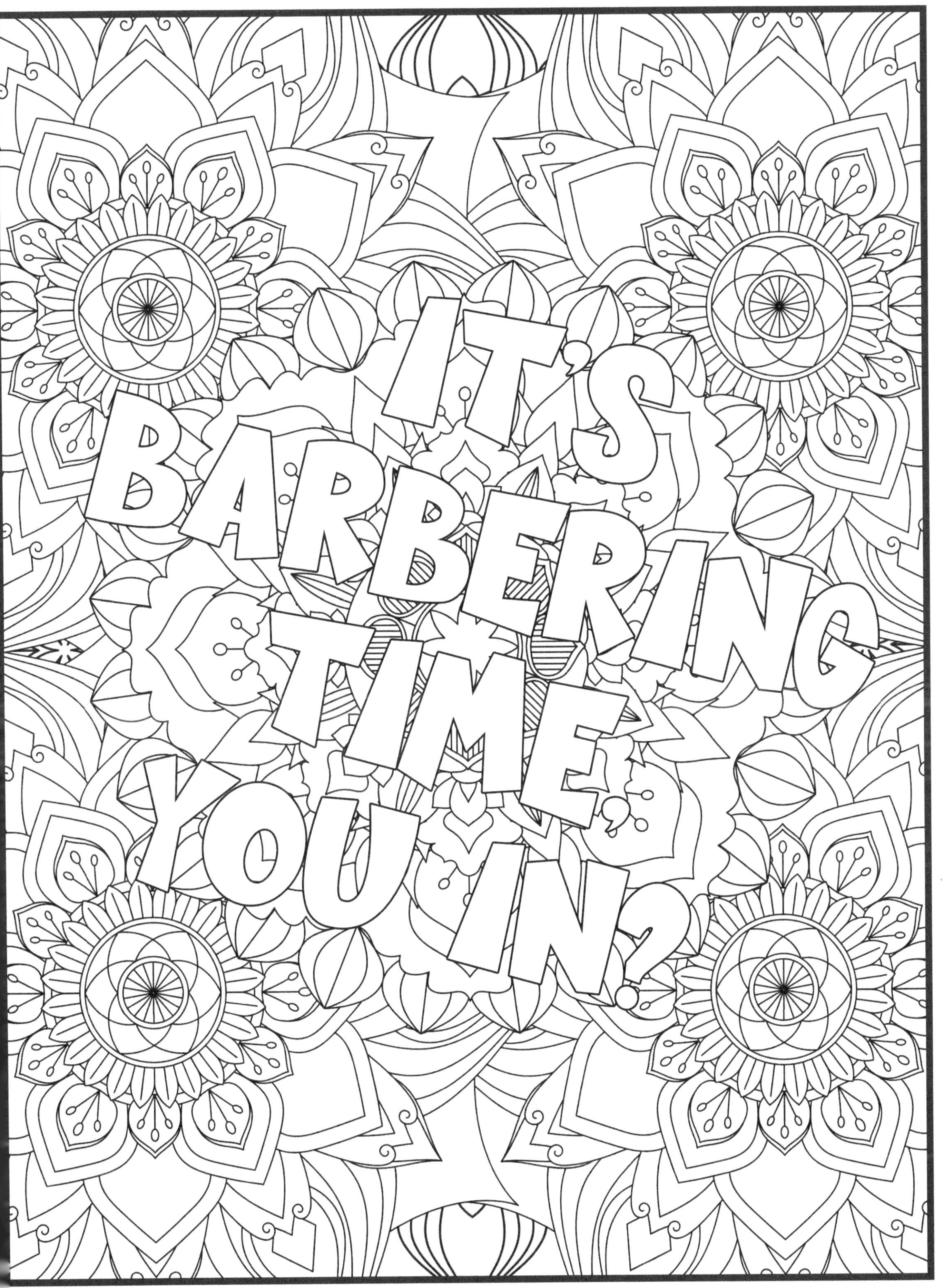

IT'S
BARBERING
TIME,
YOU IN?

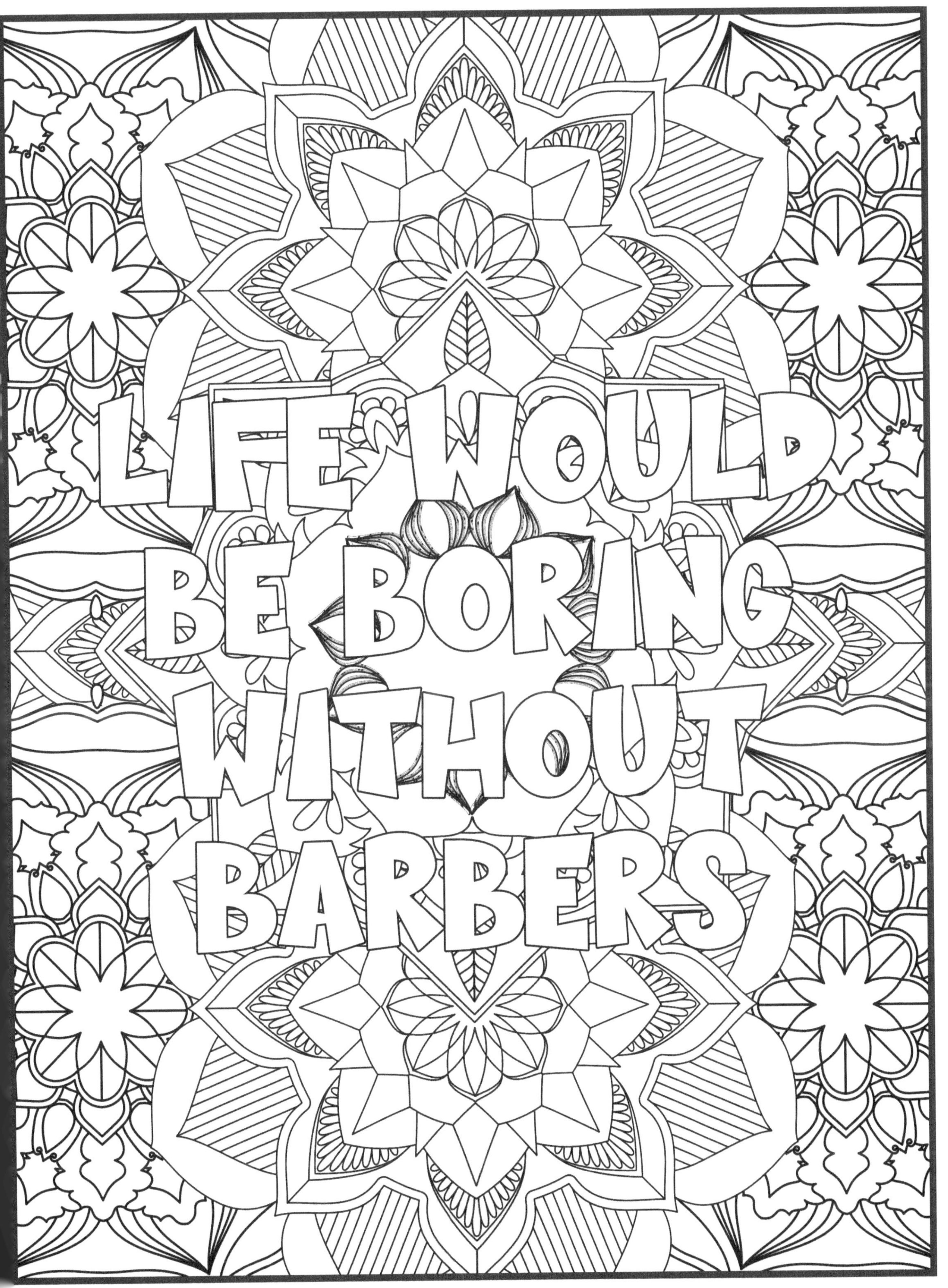

LIFE WOULD
BE BORING
WITHOUT
BARBERS

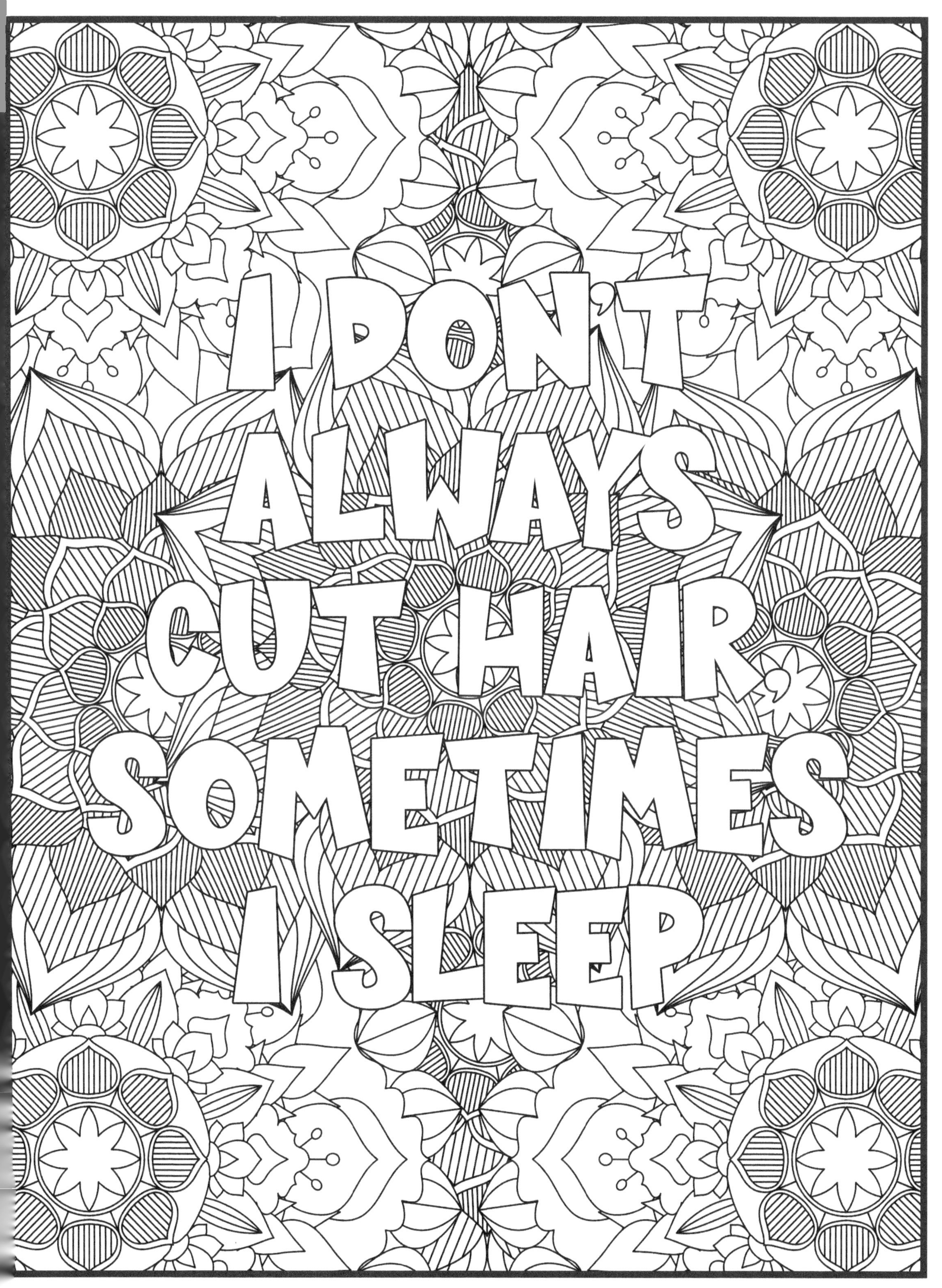

I DON'T
ALWAYS
CUT HAIR,
SOMETIMES
I SLEEP

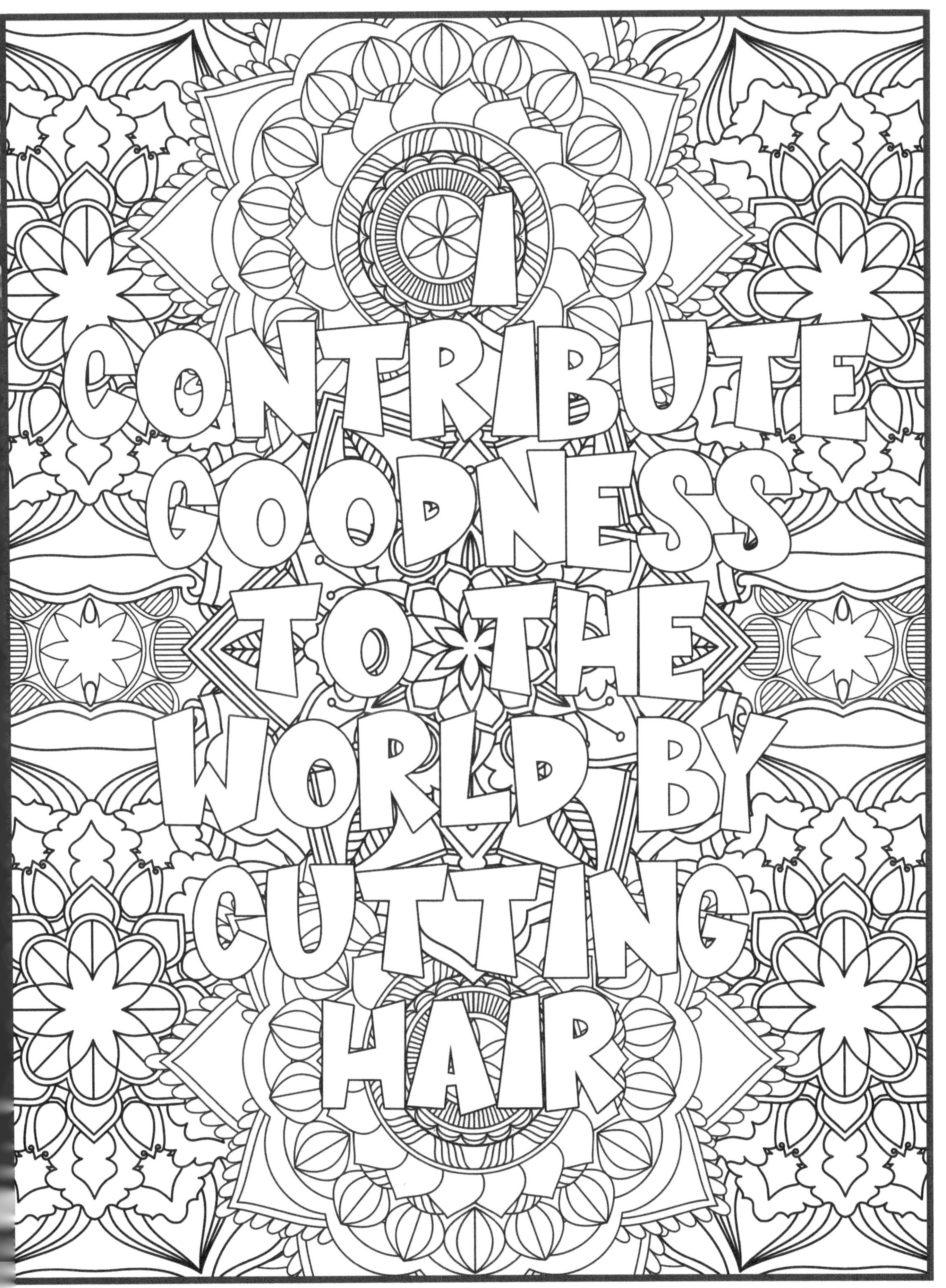

I CONTRIBUTE GOODNESS TO THE WORLD BY CUTTING HAIR

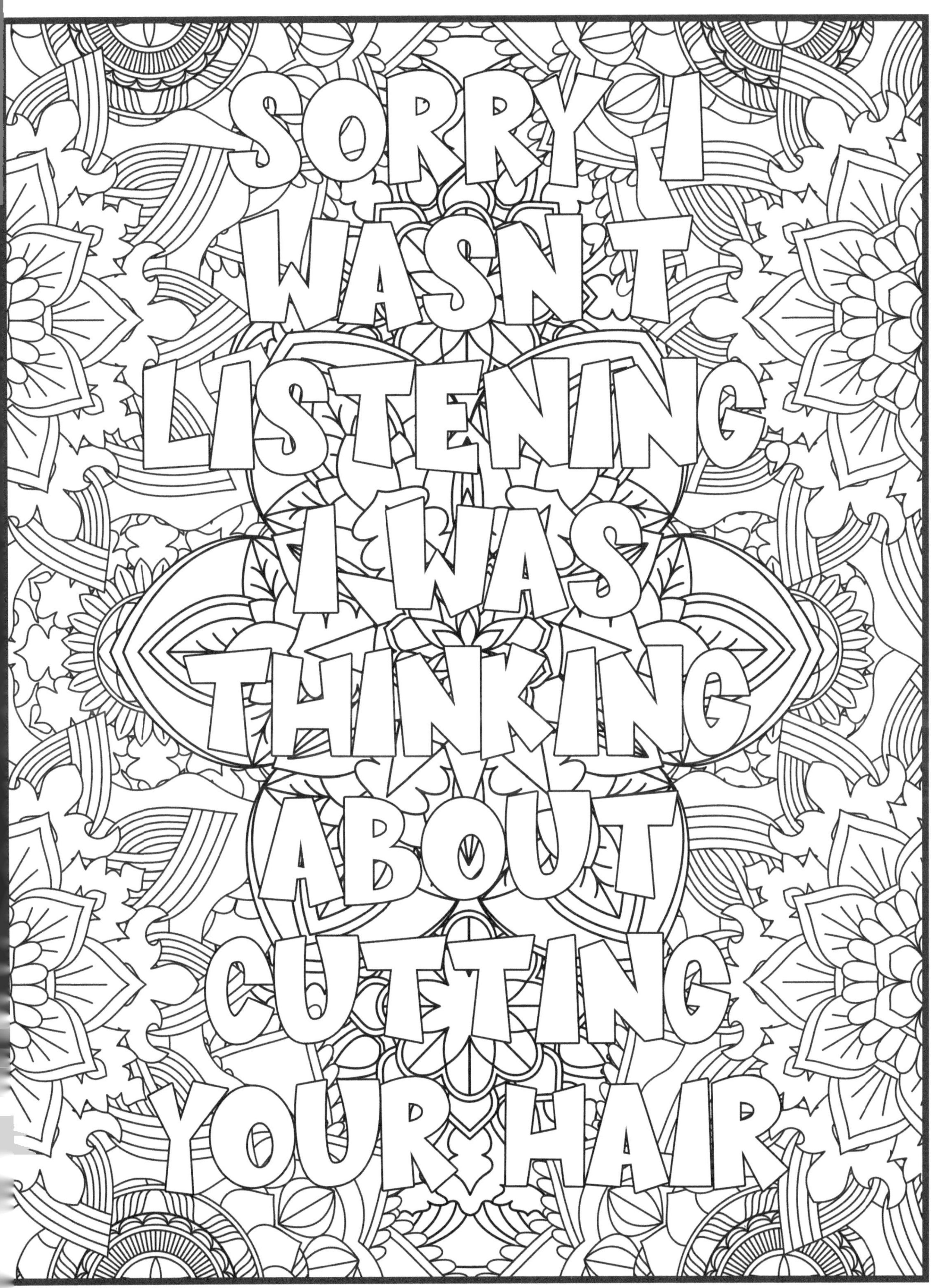

SORRY I
WASN'T
LISTENING
I WAS
THINKING
ABOUT
CUTTING
YOUR HAIR

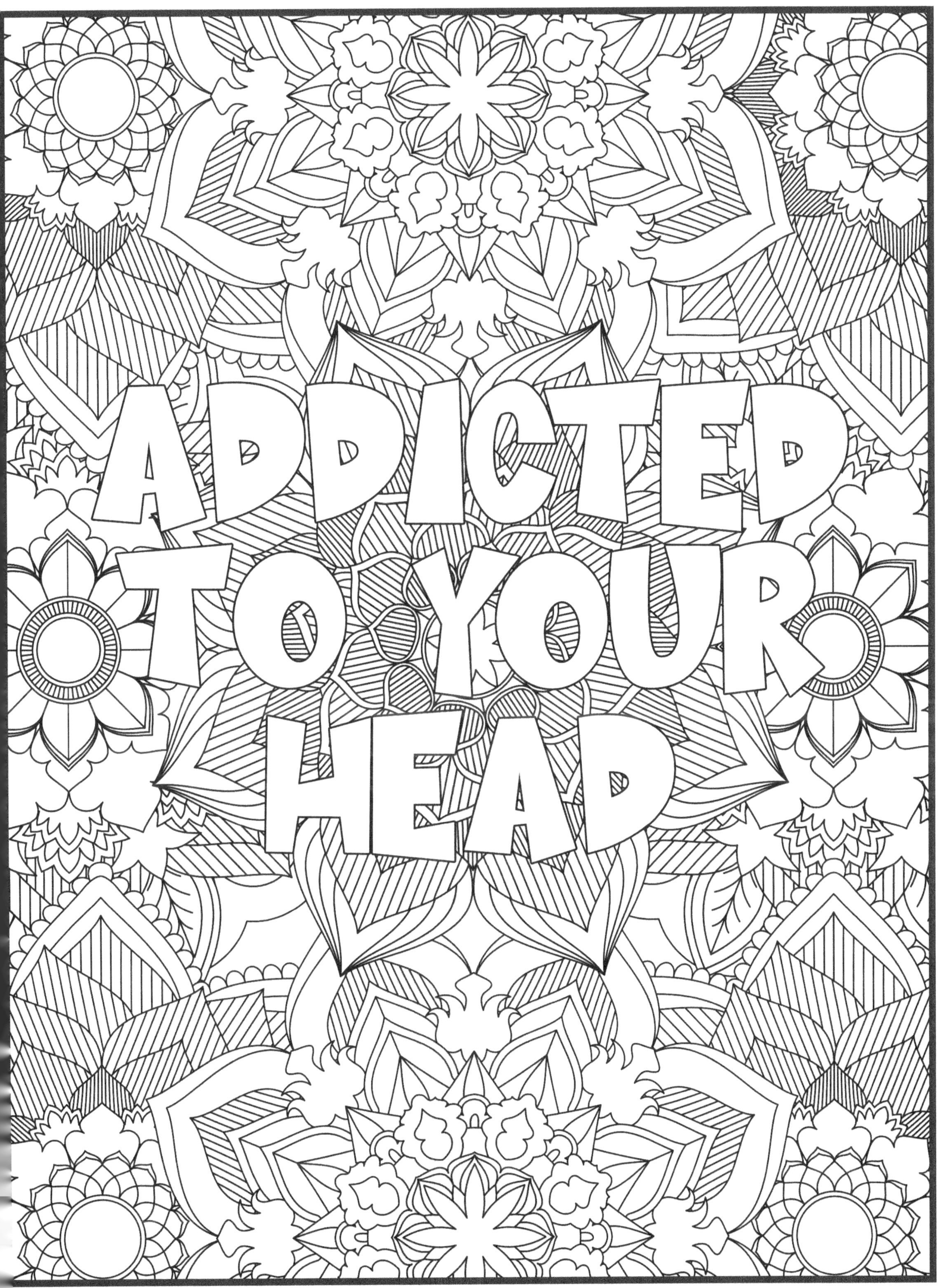
ADDICTED TO YOUR HEAD

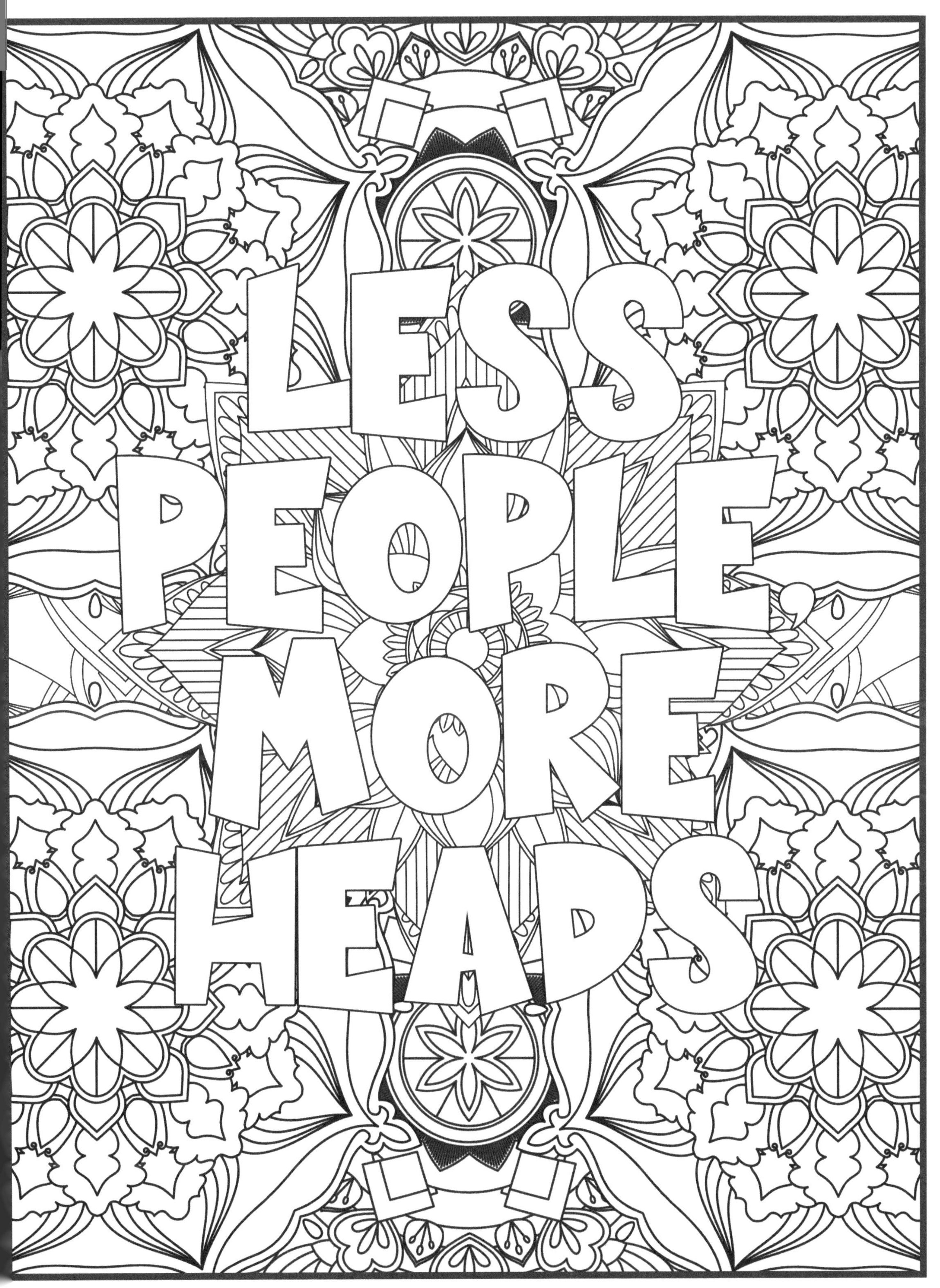

LESS PEOPLE,
MORE HEADS

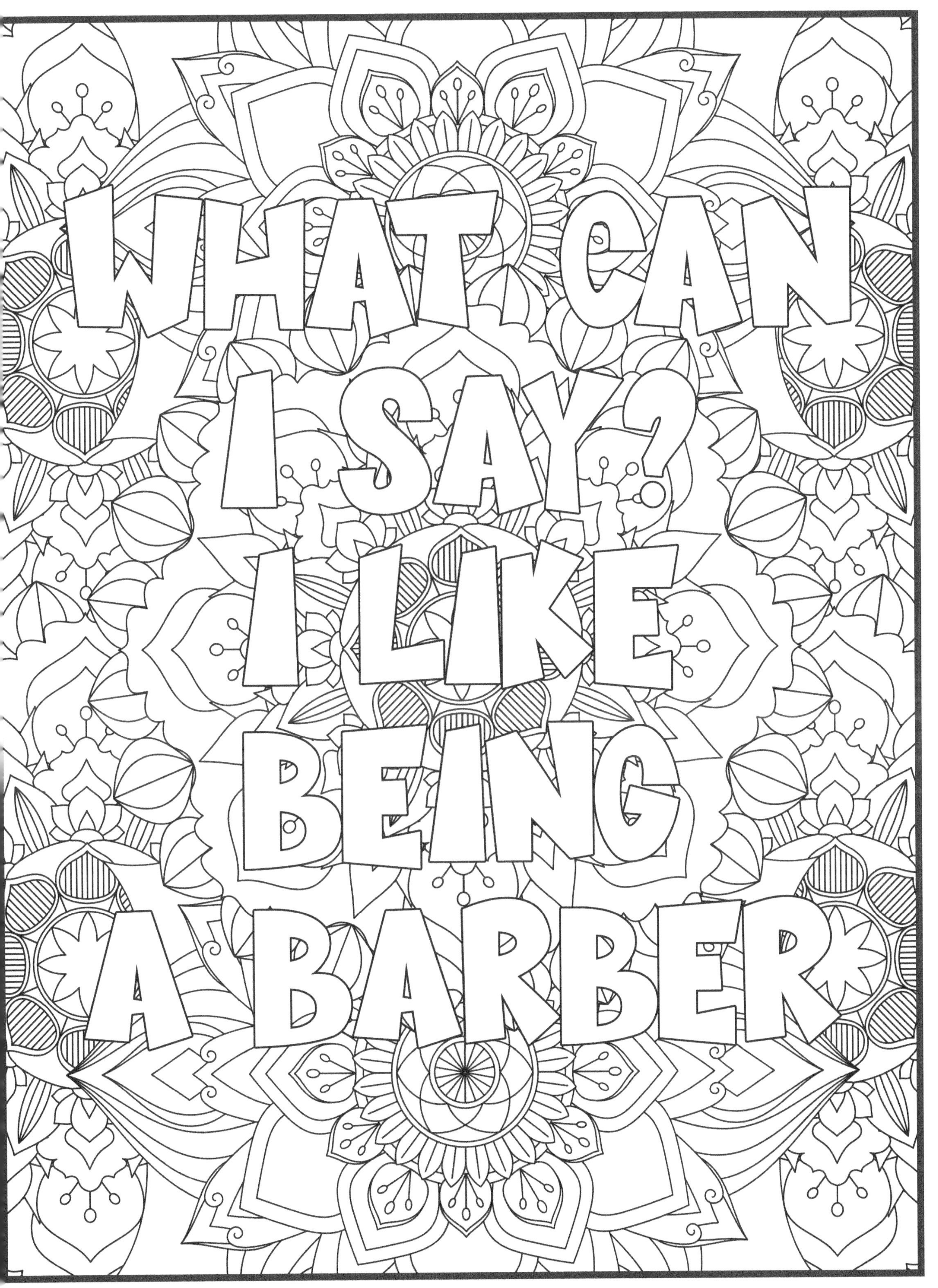

WHAT CAN
I SAY?
I LIKE
BEING
A BARBER

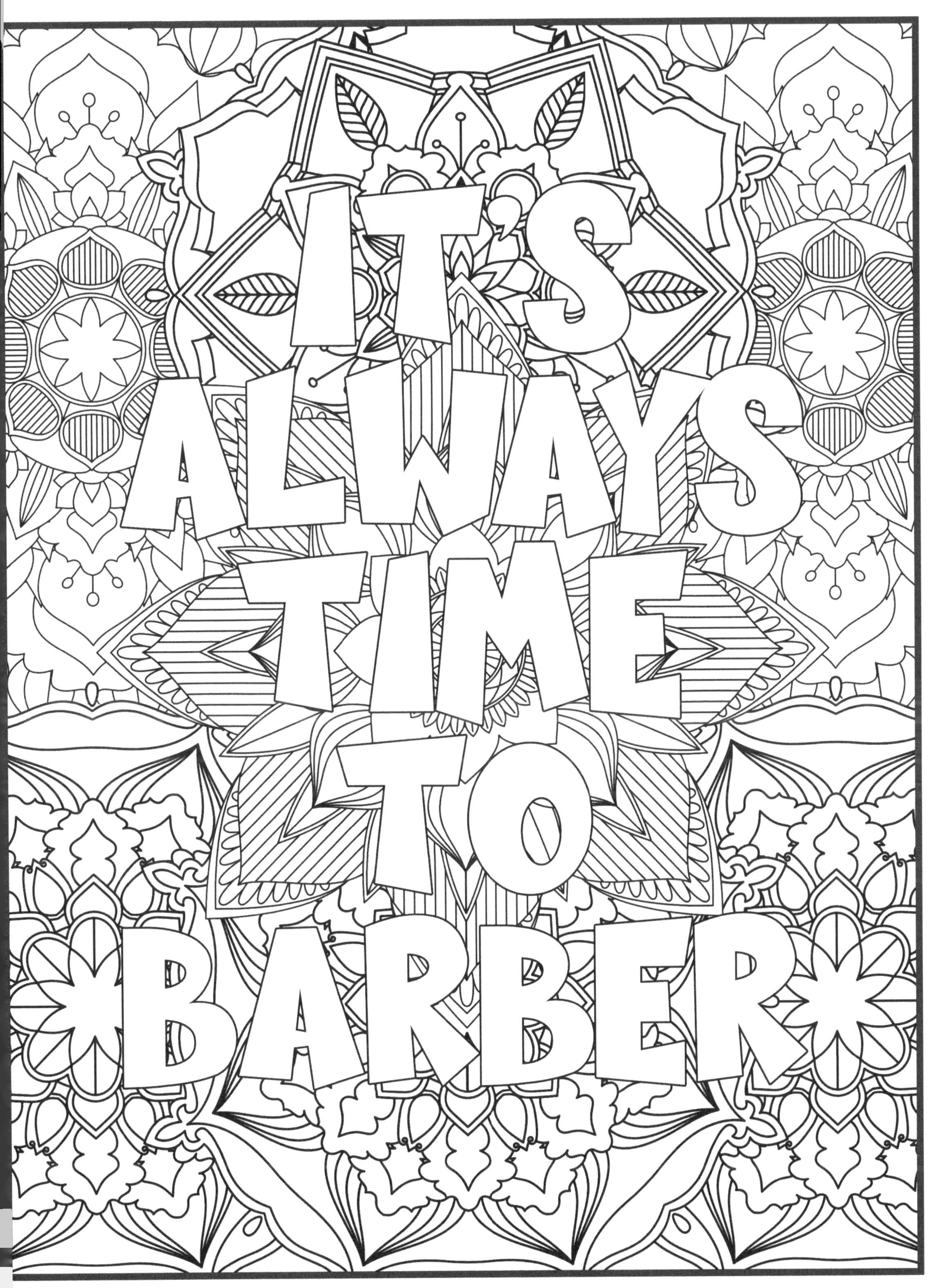
IT'S
ALWAYS
TIME
TO
BARBER

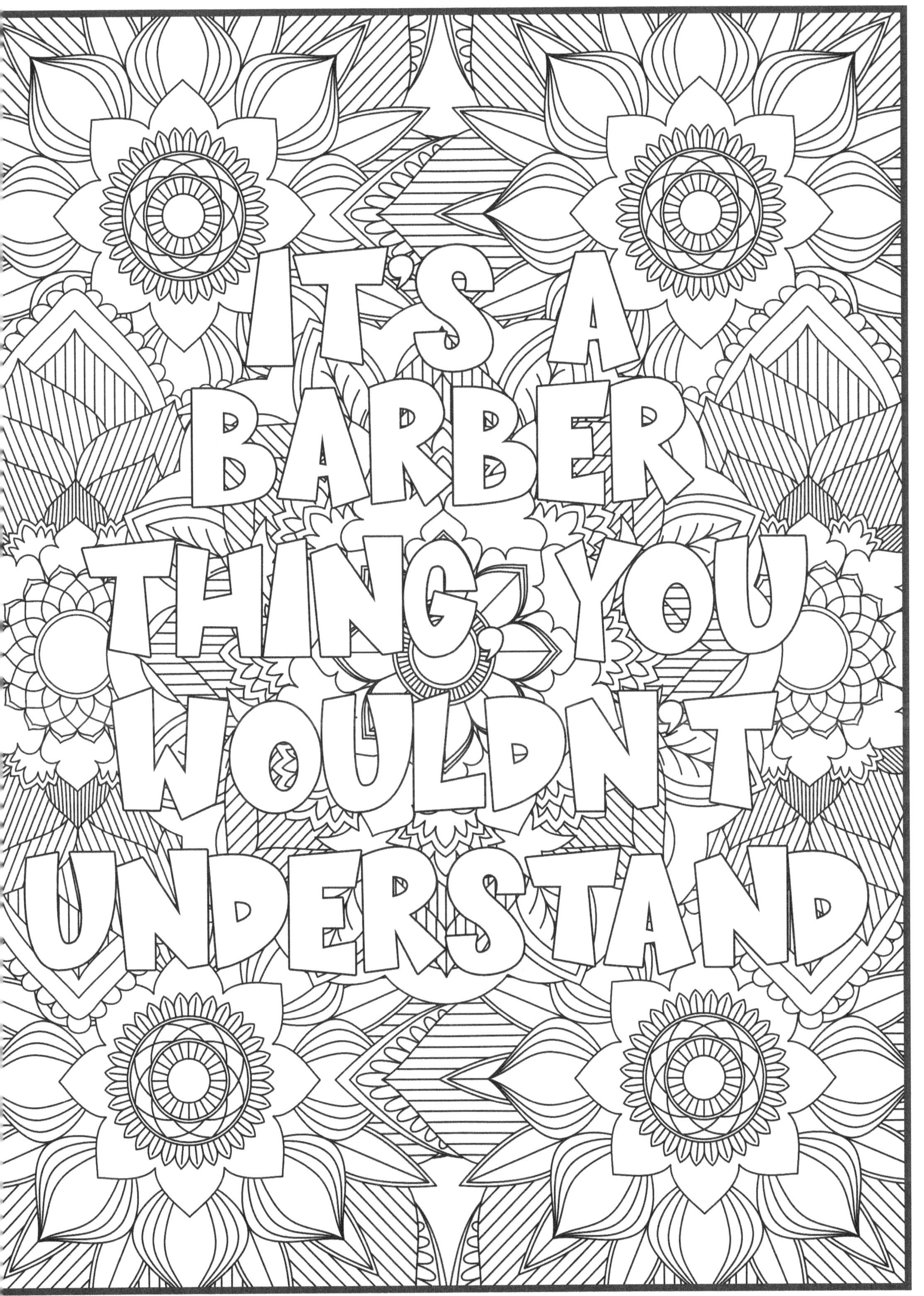

IT'S A
BARBER
THING, YOU
WOULDN'T
UNDERSTAND

www.ingramcontent.com/pod-product-compliance
Lightning Source LLC
Chambersburg PA
CBHW081457250726
48662CB00009B/3131